Mediterranean Lunch & Dinner Recipes

Simple and Quick Mediterranean Recipes for Lunches and Dinners

Ben Cooper

Table of contents

Tuna, Egg & Caper Salad

Preparation Time: 5 Minutes
Cooking Time: 20 Minutes
Servings: 2

Ingredients:

100g 3½oz. red chicory or yellow if not available
150g 5oz tinned tuna flakes in brine, drained
100g 3 ½ oz. cucumber
25g 1oz rocket arugula pitted black olives
hard-boiled eggs, peeled and quartered tomatoes, chopped
1 tablespoons fresh parsley, chopped
1 red onion, chopped
1 stalk of celery
1 tablespoon capers
2 tablespoons garlic vinaigrette

Directions:

1.Place the tuna, cucumber, olives, tomatoes, onion, chicory, celery, parsley, and rocket arugula into a bowl.

2.Serve onto plates and scatter the eggs and capers on top.

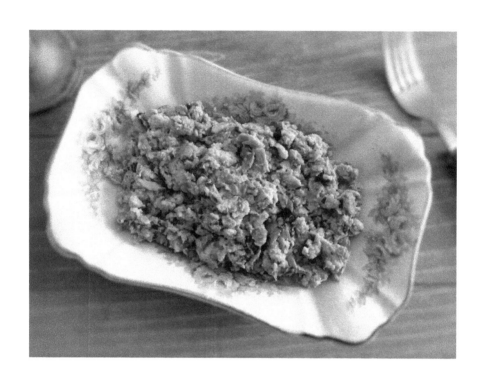

Salmon and Capers

Preparation Time: 10 minutes
Cooking Time: 0
Servings: 4

Ingredients:

75g (3oz) Greek yogurt salmon fillets, skin removed
1 tsp Dijon Mustard
1 tbsp capers, chopped
1 tsp fresh parsley
Zest of 1 lemon

Directions:

1.In a bowl, mix the yogurt, mustard, lemon zest, parsley and capers.

2.Thoroughly coat the salmon in the mixture.

3.Place the salmon under a hot grill (broiler) and cook for 3-4 minutes on each side, or until the fish is cooked.

4.Serve with mashed potatoes and vegetables or a large green leafy salad.

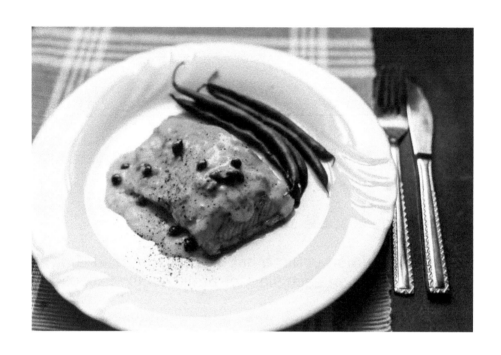

Rocket salad with Tuna

Preparation Time: 5 minutes
Cooking Time: 15 minutes
Servings: 4

Ingredients:

Slices rustic bread, torn into pieces large tomatoes
1 Tbsp. olive oil
400g tin cannellini beans, drained and rinsed
¼ cup Kalamata olives cups shredded rocket
¼ red onion, sliced finely
85g tin tuna

Dressing:

Tbsp. olive oil
½ tsp. dijon mustard
1 Tbsp. lemon juice

Directions:

1.Start with setting the oven at 180C.

2.Place the bread slices in braking tray, put olive oil on slices and bake for 10-15 mins.

3.To prepare the dressing mix lemon juice, mustard and oil in a jar.

4.Bring a bowl, add baked bread, onions, beans, tuna, tomatoes and rocket.

6.Put the dressing over salad and enjoy.

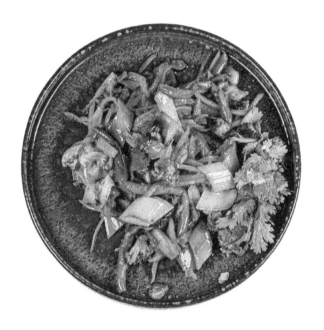

Sirt Super Salad

Preparation Time: 5 minutes
Cooking Time: 15 minutes
Servings: 1

Ingredients:

1 3/4 ounces (50g) arugula
1/2 ounces (100g) smoked salmon slices
1 3/4 ounces (50g) endive leaves
1/2 cup (50g) celery including leaves, sliced
1/8 cups (15g) walnuts, chopped
1/2 cup (80g) avocado, peeled, stoned, and sliced
1/8 cup (20g) red onion, sliced
1 tablespoon extra-virgin olive oil
1 tablespoon capers
1 large Medjool date, pitted and chopped
1/4 cup (10g) parsley, chopped
Juice of 1/4 lemon

Directions:

1.Bring a bowl, place large leaves of salad, add all the ingredients one by one in the bowl and stir through the bowl and enjoy.

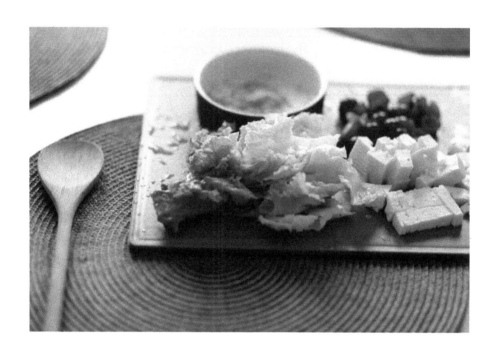

Strawberry Buckwheat Tabbouleh

Preparation Time: 5 minutes
Cooking Time: 15 minutes
Servings: 1

Ingredients:

1/3 cup (50g) buckwheat
1/2 cup (80g) avocado
1 tablespoon ground turmeric
1/8 cup (20g) red onion
3/8 cup (65g) tomato
1 tablespoon capers
1/8 cup (25g) Medjool dates, pitted
2/3 cup (100g) strawberries, hulled
3/4 cup (30g) parsley
1 tablespoon extra-virgin olive oil
1 ounce (30g) arugula
Juice of 1/2 lemon

Directions:

1.Start with cooking the buckwheat by mixing the turmeric according to the instructions of package. Drain and let it cool.

2.Now, start chopping the tomatoes, capers, onions, avocados, dates and parsley. Mix all of them with already cooked buckwheat.

3.After that, take the strawberries, slice them and add them in salad. Garnish the salad on the arugula bed.

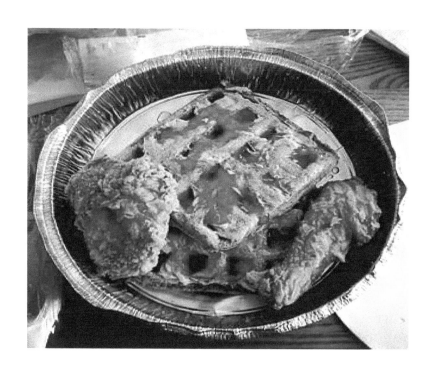

Fragrant Anise Hotpot Sirtfood

Preparation Time: 2 minutes
Cooking Time: 10 minutes
Servings: 2

Ingredients:

1 tbsp. tomato purée
1 star anise, crushed (or 1/4 tsp ground anise)
Small handful (10g) parsley, stalks finely chopped
Small handful (1Og) coriander, stalks finely chopped
Juice of 1/2 lime
1/2 carrot, peeled and cut into matchsticks
500ml chicken stock, fresh or made with 1 cube 50g
beansprouts
1OOg firm tofu, chopped
50g broccoli, cut into small florets
1OOg raw tiger prawns
50g cooked water chestnuts, drained
50g rice noodles, cooked according to packet
instructions
1 tbsp. good-quality miso paste
20g sushi ginger, chopped

Directions:

1.Take a pan and put the parsley stalks, lime juice, tomato purée, coriander stalks, star anise, and chicken stock, let them simmer for 10-12 mins.

2.Now add the broccoli, tofu, carrot, water, chestnuts, and prawns, gently mix them and let them cook completely.

3.Turn off the heat and add in the miso paste and sushi ginger.

4.Garnish with coriander and parsley leaves and enjoy.

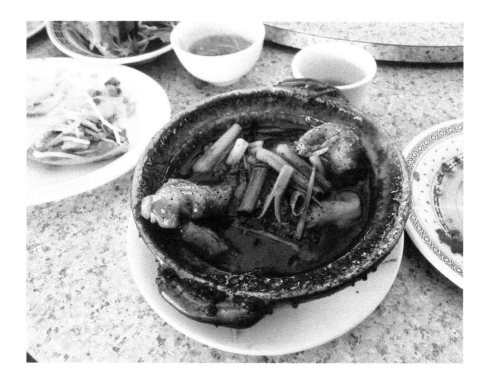

Coronation Chicken Salad Sirtfood

Preparation Time: 2 minutes
Cooking Time: 2 minutes
Servings: 1

Ingredients:

75 g Natural yoghurt
1 tsp. Coriander, chopped Juice of
1/4 of a lemon
1/2 tsp. Mild curry powder
1 tsp. Ground turmeric
Walnut halves, finely chopped
100 g Cooked chicken breast, cut into bite-sized pieces
20 g Red onion, diced
1 Bird's eye chili
1 Medjool date, finely chopped
40 g Rocket, to serve

Directions:

1.Take a bowl, gather the ingredients, mix them in bowl, and serve the salad on the rocket bedding.

Buckwheat Pasta Salad

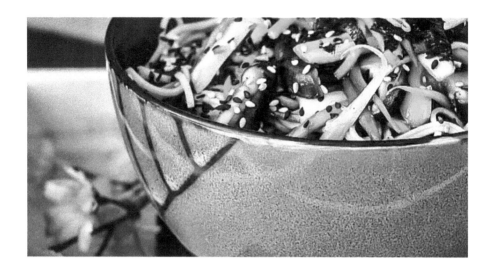

Preparation Time: 15 minutes
Cooking Time: 0 minutes
Servings: 1

Ingredients:

50g cooked buckwheat pasta small handful of basil
leaves large handful of rockets
1/2 avocado, diced
1 tbsp. extra virgin olive oil
20g pine nuts
cherry tomatoes, halved olives

Directions:

1.Take a bowl or a plate, add in all the ingredients, now
scatter the pine nuts all over the ingredients and serve.

Shrimp Pasta

Preparation Time: 45 minutes
Cooking Time: 10 minutes
Servings: 2

Ingredients:
ounces linguine
¼ cup mayonnaise
¼ cup bean stew glue
Two cloves garlic, squashes
½ pound shrimp, stripped
1 teaspoon salt
½ teaspoon cayenne pepper
1 teaspoon garlic powder
1.tablespoon vegetable oil
One lime, squeezed
¼ cup green onion, slashed
¼ cup cilantro, minced
Red bean stew chips, for embellish

Directions:

1.Cook pasta still somewhat firm as per box guidelines. In a little bowl, consolidate mayonnaise, stew glue and garlic. Race to join. Put in a safe spot. In a blending bowl, include shrimp, salt, cayenne and garlic powder.

2.Mix to cover shrimp. Oil in a heavy skillet over medium warmth. Include shrimp and cook for around 2 minutes to flip and cook for an extra 2 minutes.

3. Add pasta and sauce to the dish. Mood killer the warmth and combine until the pasta is covered.

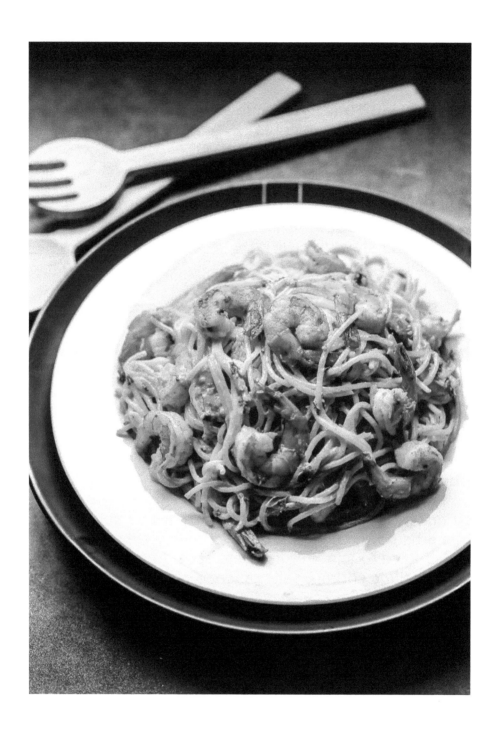

Chicken Thighs with Creamy Tomato Spinach Sauce

Preparation Time: 45 minutes
Cooking Time: 10 minutes
Servings: 2

Ingredients:

1 tablespoon olive oil
lb. chicken thighs, boneless skinless
½ teaspoon salt
¼ teaspoon pepper oz. tomato sauce
Two garlic cloves, minced
½ cup overwhelming cream oz. new spinach
Four leaves fresh basil (or utilize ¼ teaspoon dried basil)

Directions:

1.The most effective method to cook boneless skinless chicken thighs in a skillet: In a much skillet heat olive oil on medium warmth. Boneless chicken with salt and pepper. Add top side down to the hot skillet.

2.Cook for 5 minutes on medium heat, until the high side, is pleasantly burned. Flip over to the opposite side and heat for five additional minutes on medium heat. Expel the chicken from the skillet to a plate.

3.Step by step instructions to make creamy tomato basil sauce: To the equivalent, presently void skillet, include tomato sauce, minced garlic, and substantial cream. Bring to bubble and mix. Lessen warmth to low stew. Include new spinach and new basil. Mix until spinach withers and diminishes in volume.

23

4.Taste the sauce and include progressively salt and pepper, if necessary. Include back cooked boneless skinless chicken thighs, increment warmth to medium.

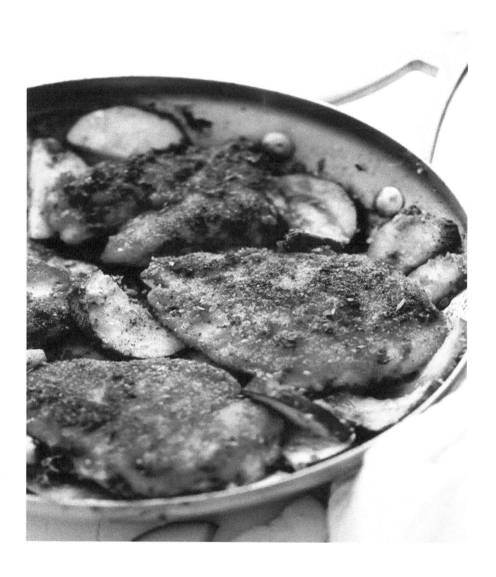

Prawn & Chili Pak Choi

Preparation Time: 30 minutes
Cooking Time: 15 minutes
Servings: 1

Ingredients:

75g (2 ¼ oz.) brown rice
1 pak choi
60ml (2 fl. oz.) chicken stock
1 tbsp. extra virgin olive oil
1 garlic clove, finely chopped
50g (1 ⅝ oz.) red onion, finely chopped
½ bird's eye chili, finely chopped
1 tsp freshly grated ginger
125g (4 ¼ oz.) shelled raw king prawns
1 tbsp. soy sauce
1 tsp five-spice
1 tbsp. freshly chopped flat-leaf parsley
A pinch of salt and pepper

Directions:

1.Bring a medium-sized saucepan of water to the boil and cook the brown rice for 25-30 minutes, or until softened.

2.Tear the pak choi into pieces. Warm the chicken stock in a skillet over medium heat and toss in the pak choi, cooking until the pak choi has slightly wilted.

3.In another skillet, warm olive oil over high heat. Toss in the ginger, chili, red onions and garlic frying for 2-3 minutes.

4.Throw in the prawns, five-spice and soy sauce and cook for 6-8 minutes, or until the cooked throughout. Drain the brown rice and add to the skillet, stirring and cooking for 2-3 minutes. Add the pak choi, garnish with parsley and serve.

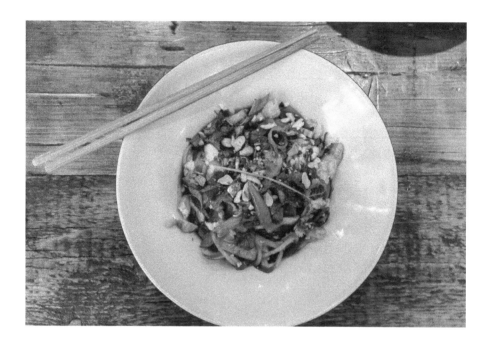

Dahl with Kale, Red Onions and Buckwheat

Preparation Time: 5 Minutes
Cooking Time: 20 Minutes
Servings: 2

Ingredients:
1 teaspoon of extra virgin olive oil
1 teaspoon of mustard seeds
40g (1 ½ oz.) red onions, finely chopped
1 clove of garlic, very finely chopped
1 teaspoon very finely chopped ginger
1 Thai chili, very finely chopped
1 teaspoon curry mixture teaspoons turmeric
300ml (10 fl. oz.) vegetable broth
40g (1 ½ oz.) red lentils
50g (1 ⅝ oz.) kale, chopped
50ml (1.70 fl. oz.) coconut milk
50g (1 ⅝ oz.) buckwheat

Directions:

1.Heat oil in a pan at medium temperature and add mustard seeds. When they crack, add onion, garlic, ginger and chili. Heat until everything is soft.

2.Add the curry powder and 1 teaspoon of turmeric, mix well.

3.Add the lentils and cook them for 25 to 30 minutes until they are ready.

4.While the lentils are cooking, prepare the buckwheat.

5.Serve buckwheat with the dal.

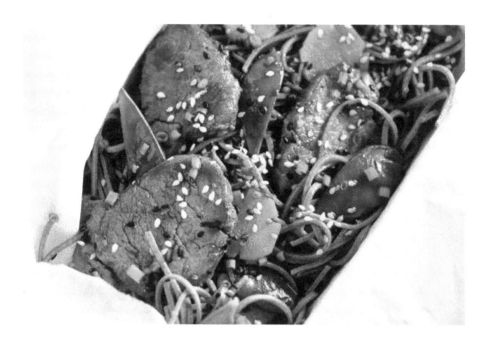

Chickpeas, Onion, Tomato & Parsley Salad in a Jar

Preparation Time: 5 Minutes

Cooking Time: 50 Minutes

Servings: 2

Ingredients:

1 cup cooked chickpeas
½ cup chopped tomatoes
½ of a small onion, chopped 1 tbsp. chia seeds
1 Tbsp. chopped parsley Dressing:
1 tbsp. olive oil and 1 tbsp. of Chlorella.
1 tbsp. fresh lemon juice and a pinch of sea salt

Directions:

1.Put ingredients in this order: dressing, tomatoes, chickpeas, onions and parsley.

Kale & Feta Salad with Cranberry Dressing

Preparation Time: 5 Minutes
Cooking Time: 30 Minutes
Servings: 2

Ingredients:
9oz kale, finely chopped
2oz walnuts, chopped
3oz feta cheese, crumbled
1 apple, peeled, cored and sliced medjool dates, chopped
For the Dressing 3oz cranberries
½ red onion, chopped tablespoons olive oil
1 tablespoons water teaspoons honey
1 tablespoon red wine vinegar Sea salt

Directions:

1.Place the ingredients for the dressing into a food processor and process until smooth. If it seems too thick, you can add a little extra water if necessary. Place all the ingredients for the salad into a bowl.

2.Pour on the dressing and toss the salad until it is well coated in the mixture.

Spiced Fish Tacos with Fresh Corn Salsa

Preparation Time: 10 minutes
Cooking Time: 20 minutes
Servings: 4

Ingredients:
1 cup corn
1/2 cup red onion, diced
1 cup jicama, peeled and chopped
1/2 cup red bell pepper, diced
1 cup fresh cilantro leaves, finely chopped
1 lime, zested and juiced
1 tablespoons sour cream tablespoons cayenne pepper
Salt and pepper to taste
(4 ounce) fillets tilapia tablespoons olive oil corn tortillas, warmed

Directions:

1.If you do not have any available, you can substitute for water chestnuts, celery, or radishes.

2.Preheat grill for high heat.

For the Corn Salsa:

1.In a medium bowl, mix corn, red onion, jicama, red bell pepper, and cilantro. Stir in lime juice and zest.

2.Brush each fillet with olive oil, and sprinkle with the cayenne and season to taste.

3.Arrange fillets on the grill and cook for 3 minutes per side. For each fish taco, top two corn tortillas with fish, sour cream, and corn salsa.

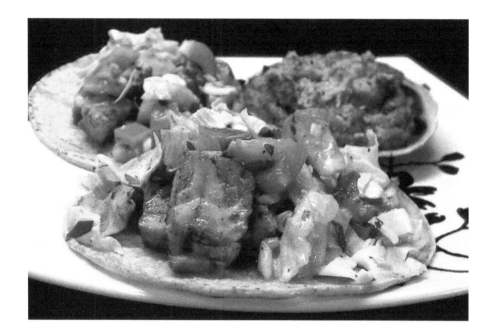

Sautee Tofu & Kale

Preparation Time: 10 minutes
Cooking Time: 10 minutes
Servings: 3

Ingredients:
12 oz. extra firm tofu tbsps. olive oil
½ tsp. salt & pepper
1 tsp. garlic, minced
1 bunch kale, chopped

Directions:

1.Heat oil in a large skillet over medium heat.

2.Fry tofu in a pan for 4-5 minutes.

3.Add kale and stir fry for 3-4 minutes until kale is soft.

4.Add salt, pepper and garlic, and cook for another 1-2 minutes until the garlic is fragrant.

5.Drizzle sesame seeds on top.

6.Serve and enjoy!

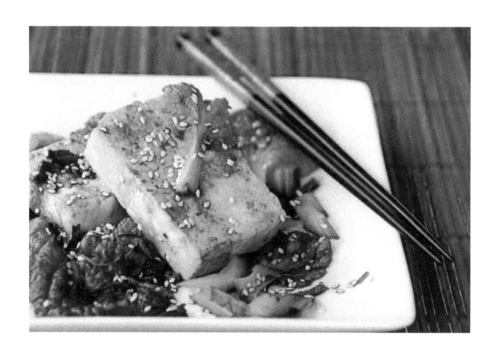

Chicken and Lentil Stew

Preparation Time: 10 minutes
Cooking Time: 40 minutes
Servings: 3

Ingredients:
Chicken breasts, diced
½ cup red lentils, rinsed
1 carrot, chopped
1 small onion, chopped
1 garlic clove, chopped
1 celery stalk, chopped
1 small red pepper, chopped
1 can tomatoes, chopped
1 tbsp. paprika
1 tsp ginger, grated
tbsp. extra virgin olive oil
½ cup fresh parsley leaves, finely cut, to serve

Directions:

1.Heat olive oil in a casserole and gently brown the chicken, stirring.

2.Add in onions, garlic, celery, carrot, pepper, paprika and ginger.

3.Cook, constantly stirring, for 2-3 minutes.

4.Add in the lentils and tomatoes and bring to a boil.

5.Lower heat, cover, and simmer for 30 minutes, or until the lentils are tender and the chicken is cooked through.

6.Serve sprinkled with fresh parsley

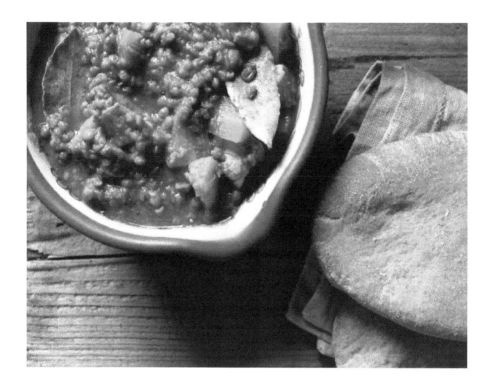

Mussels in Red Wine Sauce

Preparation Time: 10 minutes
Cooking Time: 25 minutes
Servings: 2

Ingredients:

800g (2lb) mussels
400g (14oz) tins of chopped tomatoes
25g (1oz) butter
1 tablespoon fresh chives, chopped
1 tablespoon fresh parsley, chopped
1 bird's-eye chilli, finely chopped cloves of garlic, crushed
400mls (14fl oz.) red wine Juice of 1 lemon

Directions:

1.Wash the mussels, remove their beards and set them aside.

2.Heat the butter in a large saucepan and add in the red wine. Reduce the heat and add the parsley, chives, chilli and garlic while stirring.

3.Add in the tomatoes, lemon juice and mussels. Cover the saucepan and cook for 2-3.Remove the saucepan from the heat and take out any mussels which haven't opened and discard them.

4.Serve and eat immediately.

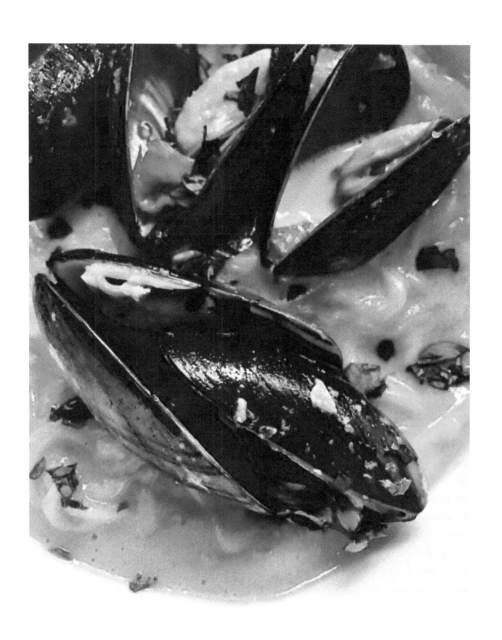

Breakfast Salad from Grains and Fruits

Preparation Time: 15 minutes
Cooking Time: 20 minutes
Servings: 6

Ingredients:

¼ tsp. salt
¾ cup bulgur
¾ cup quick cooking brown rice
1 8-oz. low fat vanilla yogurt
1 cup raisins
1 Granny Smith apple
1 orange
1 Red delicious apple
3 cups water

Directions:

1.On high fire, place a large pot and bring water to a boil.

2.Add bulgur and rice. Lower fire to a simmer and cook for ten minutes while covered.

3.Turn off fire, set aside for 2 minutes while covered. In baking sheet, transfer and evenly spread grains to cool. Meanwhile, peel oranges and cut into sections. Chop and core apples.

4.Once grains are cool, transfer to a large serving bowl along with fruits. Add yogurt and mix well to coat.

5.Serve and enjoy.

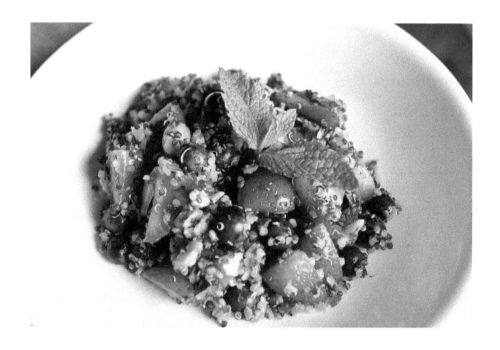

Delicious Rice and Spinach

Preparation Time: 10 minutes
Cooking Time: 15 minutes
Servings: 6

Ingredients:

1 onion
2 pinch sea salt
2 pinch black pepper.
1 cup unsalted vegetable broth
2 tablespoons olive oil.
2 can brown rice
4 cups fresh baby spinach
Juice of orange
1 garlic clove
1 orange Zest

Directions:

1.In a substantial skillet over medium-high heat the olive oil until it gleams. Include the onion and for around 5 minutes blending infrequently until delicate.

2.Include the spinach and for around 2 minutes blending infrequently until it fades.

3.Include the garlic and for 30 seconds blending continually. Blend in the orange juice soup ocean salt and pepper. Convey to a stew.

4.Mix in the rice and for around 4 minutes mixing until the rice is warmed through and the fluid is consumed.

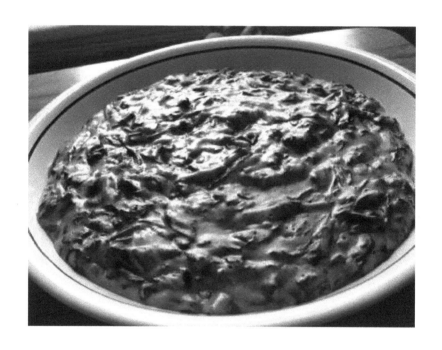

Blue Cheese and Grains Salad

Preparation Time: 15 minutes
Cooking Time: 40 minutes
Servings: 4

Ingredients:

¼ cup thinly sliced scallions
½ cup millet, rinsed
½ cup quinoa, rinsed
1 ½ tsp. olive oil
1 garlic, minced Oz. blue cheese
2 tbsp. fresh lemon juice
2 tsp. dried rosemary
4-oz. boneless, skinless chicken breasts
6 oz. baby spinach olive oil cooking spray

Dressing ingredients:
¼ cup fresh raspberries
1 tbsp. pure maple syrup
1 tsp. fresh thyme leaf
2 tbsp. grainy mustard
6 tbsp. balsamic vinegar

Directions:

1.Bring millet, quinoa, and 2 ¼ cups water on a small saucepan to a boil. Once boiling, slow fire to a simmer and stir.

2.Cover and cook until water is fully absorbed and grains are soft around 15 minutes.

3.Turn off fire, fluff grains with a fork and set aside to cool a bit.

Arrange one oven rack to highest position and preheat broiler. Line a baking sheet with foil, and grease with cooking spray.

4.Whisk well pepper, oil, rosemary, lemon juice and garlic. Rub onto chicken. Place chicken on prepared pan, pop into the broiler and broil until juices run clear and no longer pin inside around 12 minutes.

5.Meanwhile, make the dressing by combining all ingredients in a blender.

6.Blend until smooth.

7.Remove chicken from oven, cool slightly before cutting into strips, against the grain.

8.To assemble, place grains in a large salad bowl. Add in dressing and spinach, toss to mix well.

9.Add scallions and pear, mix gently and evenly divide into four plates. Top each salad with cheese and chicken.

10.Serve and enjoy.

Cucumber Salad with Rice and Asparagus

Preparation Time: 15 minutes
Cooking Time: 21 minutes
Servings: 6

Ingredients:

4 heads butter lettuce
¼ cup chopped fresh dill
2 ½ tbsp. Vegetable oil
½ tsp. dry mustard
1 tbsp. white wine vinegar
1 tbsp. white sugar
2 tbsp. Dijon mustard
3 green onions, chopped
1 ½ cups English cucumber, peeled, seeded and chopped
1 lb. thin asparagus spears, trimmed and cut into 1-inch
1 cup long grain white rice
1 ¾ cups water

Directions:

1.Bring to a boil 1 ¾ cups water in a medium saucepan. Add rice and bring again to a boil. Once boiling, reduce fire to low. Continue cooking around 20 minutes or until water is fully absorbed and rice is tender.

2.Turn of fire and fluff rice with a fork and transfer to a bowl to cool.

For 1 minute, cook asparagus in boiling and salted water. Drain and rinse asparagus and cut into 1-inch long pieces.

3.Mix rice, green onions, cucumber and asparagus thoroughly. Cover and chill In a separate medium bowl, stir thoroughly chopped dill, oil, dry mustard, vinegar, sugar and mustard. Cover and chill.

4.Mix dressing and salad and season with pepper and salt to taste.
Then, in a large bowl lined with lettuce, transfer the rice salad and garnish with dill sprigs. Serve and enjoy.

Mexican Baked Beans and Rice

Preparation Time: 30 minutes
Cooking Time: 45 minutes
Servings: 6

Ingredients:

1 ½ cups cooked brown rice
1 15-oz. can no-salt added black beans, drained and rinsed
1 cup chopped poblano pepper
1 cup chopped red bell pepper
1 cup frozen yellow corn
1 cup shredded reduced fat Monterey Jack cheese
1 lb. skinless, boneless chicken breast cut into bite sized pieces
1 tbsp. chili powder
1 tbsp. cumin
2 14.5-oz. cans no salt added tomatoes, diced or crushed
4 garlic cloves, crushed

Directions:

1.With cooking spray, grease a 3-quart shallow casserole and preheat oven to 400oF.

2.Spread cooked brown rice in bottom of casserole. Layer chicken on top of brown rice.

3.Mix well garlic, seasonings, peppers, corn, beans and tomatoes in a medium bowl.

4.Evenly spread bean mixture on top of chicken.
Sprinkle cheese on top of beans and pop into the oven.
Bake for 45 minutes, remove from oven and serve.

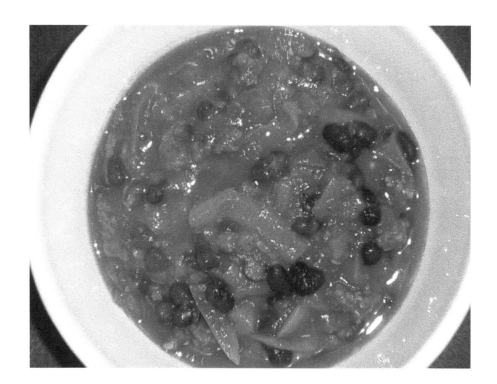

Raisins, Nuts and Beef on Hashweh Rice

Preparation Time: 20 minutes
Cooking Time: 50 minutes
Servings: 8

Ingredients:

½ cup dark raisins, soaked in 2 cups water for an hour
1/3 cup slivered almonds, toasted and soaked in 2 cups water overnight 1/3 cup pine nuts, toasted and soaked in 2 cups water overnight
½ cup fresh parsley leaves, roughly chopped pepper and salt to taste
¾ tsp. ground cinnamon, divided
¾ tsp. cloves, divided ,1 tsp. garlic powder
1 ¾ tsp. allspice, divided
1 lb. lean ground beef or lean ground lamb ,1 small red onion, finely chopped
Olive oil
1 ½ cups medium grain rice

Directions:

1.For 15 to 20 minutes, soak rice in cold water. You will know that soaking is enough when you can snap a grain of rice easily between your thumb and index finger. Once soaking is done, drain rice well.

2.Meanwhile, drain pine nuts, almonds and raisins for at least a minute and transfer to one bowl. Set aside.

3.On a heavy cooking pot on medium high fire, heat 1 tbsp. olive oil.

4.Once oil is hot, add red onions. Sauté for a minute before adding ground meat and sauté for another minute.

5.Season ground meat with pepper, salt, ½ tsp. ground cinnamon, ½ tsp. ground cloves, 1 tsp. garlic powder, and 1 ¼ tsp. allspice.
Sauté ground meat for 10 minutes or until browned and cooked fully.

6.Drain fat.

7.In same pot with cooked ground meat, add rice on top of meat.
 Season with a bit of pepper and salt. Add remaining cinnamon, ground cloves, and allspice. Do not mix.

8.Add 1 tbsp. olive oil and 2 ½ cups of water. Bring to a boil and once boiling, lower fire to a simmer. Cook while covered until liquid is fully absorbed, around 20 to 25 minutes.
Turn of fire.

9.To serve, place a large serving platter that fully covers the mouth of the pot. Place platter upside down on mouth of pot, and invert pot. The pot's inside should now rest on the platter with the rice on the bottom of the plate and ground meat on top of it.

10.Garnish the top of the meat with raisins, almonds, pine nuts, and parsley. Serve and enjoy.

Fried Rice

Preparation Time: 10 minutes
Cooking Time: 20 minutes
Servings: 4

Ingredients:

4 cups cold cooked rice
1/2 cup peas
1 medium yellow onion, diced
5 tbsp. olive oil
4 oz. frozen medium shrimp, thawed, shelled, deveined
and chopped finely 6 oz. roast pork
3 large eggs
Salt and freshly ground black pepper
1/2 tsp. cornstarch

Directions:

1.Combine the salt and ground black pepper and 1/2
tsp. cornstarch, coat the shrimp with it. Chop the
roasted pork. Beat the eggs and set aside.

2.Stir-fry the shrimp in a wok on high fire with 1 tbsp.
heated oil until pink, around 3 minutes. Set the shrimp
aside and stir fry the roasted pork briefly. Remove both
from the pan.

3.In the same pan, stir-fry the onion until soft, Stir the
peas and cook until bright green. Remove both from
pan.

4.Add 2 tbsp. oil in the same pan, add the cooked rice.
Stir and separate the individual grains.

5.Add the beaten eggs, toss the rice. Add the roasted pork, shrimp, vegetables and onion.

6.Toss everything together. Season with salt and pepper to taste.

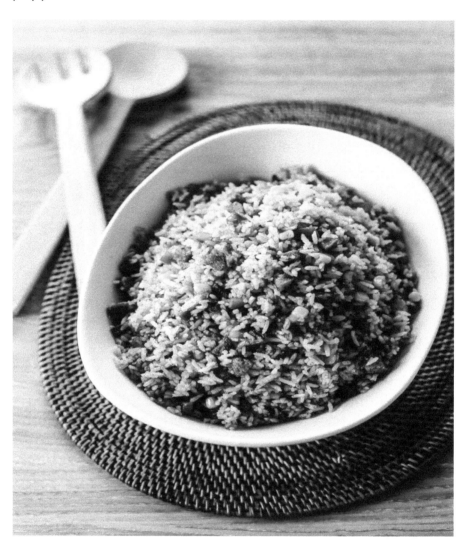

Rice & Currant Salad Mediterranean Style

Preparation Time: 30 minutes
Cooking Time: 50 minutes
Servings: 4

Ingredients:

1 cup basmati rice salt
2 1/2 Tablespoons lemon juice
1 teaspoon grated orange zest
2 Tablespoons fresh orange juice
1/4 cup olive oil
1/2 teaspoon cinnamon
Salt and pepper to taste
4 chopped green onions
1/2 cup dried currants
3/4 cup shelled pistachios or almonds
1/4 cup chopped fresh parsley

Directions:

1.Place a nonstick pot on medium high fire and add rice. Toast rice until opaque and starts to smell, around 10 minutes.

2.Add 4 quarts of boiling water to pot and 2 tsp. salt. Boil until tender, around 8 minutes uncovered.

3.Drain the rice and spread out on a lined cookie sheet to cool completely.
In a large salad bowl, whisk well the oil, juices and spices. Add salt and pepper to taste.

4.Add half of the green onions, half of parsley, currants, and nuts. Toss with the cooled rice and let stand for at least 20 minutes.

5. If needed adjust seasoning with pepper and salt. Garnish with remaining parsley and green onions.

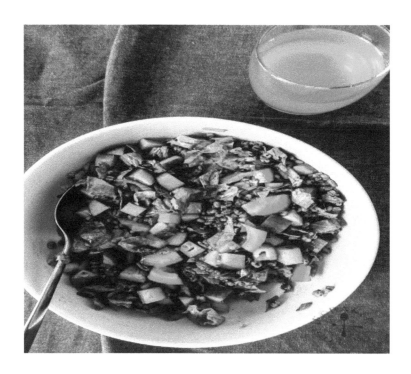

French Toast

Preparation Time: 20 minutes
Cooking Time: 10 minutes
Servings: 6

Ingredients:

1½ cups unsweetened almond milk
2 eggs, beaten
2 egg whites, beaten
1 teaspoon vanilla extract
Zest of 1 orange
Juice of 1 orange
1 teaspoon ground nutmeg
6 light whole-wheat bread slices
Nonstick cooking spray

Directions:

1.In a small bowl, whisk the almond milk, eggs, egg whites, vanilla, orange zest and juice, and nutmeg.

2.Arrange the bread in a single layer in a 9-by-13-inch baking dish. Pour the milk and egg mixture over the top. Allow the bread to soak for about 10 minutes, turning once.

3.Spray a nonstick skillet with cooking spray and heat over medium-high heat. Working in batches, add the bread and cook for about 5 minutes per side until the custard sets.

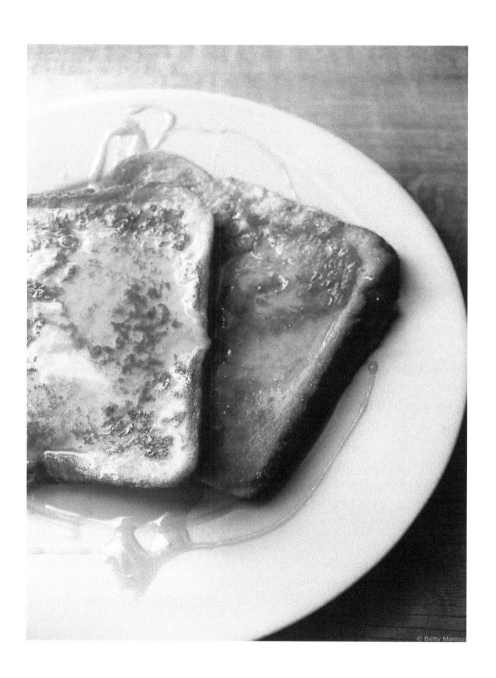
© Betty Manou

Tomato and Zucchini Frittata

Preparation Time: 10 minutes
Cooking Time: 18 minutes
Servings: 4

Ingredients:

3 eggs
3 egg whites
½ cup unsweetened almond milk
½ teaspoon sea salt
⅛ Teaspoon freshly ground black pepper
2 tablespoons extra-virgin olive oil
1 zucchini, chopped
8 cherry tomatoes, halved
¼ cup (about 2 ounces) grated Parmesan cheese

Directions:

1.Heat the oven's broiler to high, adjusting the oven rack to the center position. In a small bowl, whisk the eggs, egg whites, almond milk, sea salt, and pepper. Set aside.

2.In a 12-inch ovenproof skillet over medium-high heat, heat the olive oil until it shimmers.

3.Add the zucchini and tomatoes and cook for 5 minutes, stirring occasionally. Pour the egg mixture over the vegetables and cook for about 4 minutes without stirring until the eggs set around the edges.

4.Using a silicone spatula, pull the set eggs away from the edges of the pan. Tilt the pan in all directions to allow the unset eggs to fill the spaces along the edges.

Continue to cook for about 4 minutes more without stirring until the edges set again.

5.Sprinkle the eggs with the Parmesan. Transfer the pan to the broiler. Cook for 3 to 5 minutes until the cheese melts and the eggs are puffy. Cut into wedges to serve.

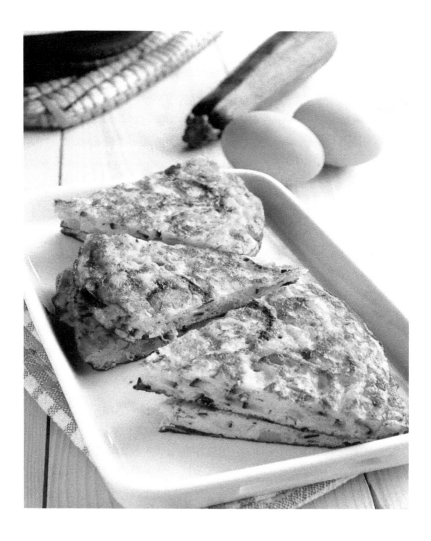

Mediterranean Pork Chops

Total time: 30Minutes
Servings: 2

Ingredients:

2 Bone-in pork chops
1 tbsp Olive oil
½ jar Ragu chunky pasta sauce
½ Red or green bell pepper

Directions:

1.Cook pork chops inside 1 of tablespoon olive oil set at medium to high heat in a 12-inch pan

2.Cook until pork chop appears brown and remove from the pan

3.Cook green pepper until it is tender using the remaining 1 tablespoon olive oil using the same pan as before, and until tender.

4.Add Pasta Sauce to the pan and set to high heat

5.Mix properly until the mixture starts to boil.

6.Set heat to low and put pork chops back into the pan.

7.Close the lid and leave to simmer for about 10 minutes or until pork is thoroughly cooked

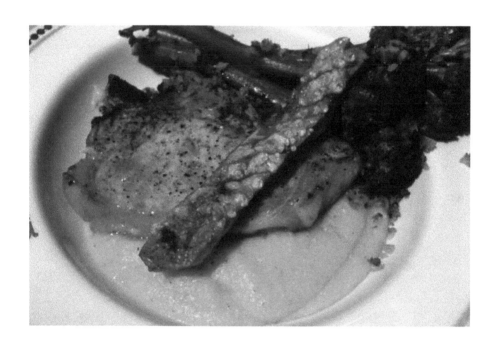

Pesto chicken pasta

Preparation time: 5 minutes
Cooking time: 20 minutes
Servings: 3

Ingredients:

2 garlic cloves
1/2 lb penne pasta
1 cup milk
1 lb boneless chicken breast
2 tbsp butter
3 oz cream cheese
1/3 cup basil pesto
1/4 cup grated Parmesan
1.5 cups chicken broth
Black pepper
1 pinch of red pepper

Directions:

1.Take the chicken breast piece & cut them into 1-inch pieces. Then add butter to a frypan & melt it.

2.Cook chicken until it turns to brown over medium heat.

3.Add the chopped garlic to it. Add garlic and chicken to the frying pan and cook it for one minute.

4.Add pasta & chicken broth to the garlic and chicken mixture.

5.Put a lid on the frypan, boil the broth on high flame.

6.After the broth is fully boiled, mix paste and heat on low flame for
eight minutes.

7.Once the pasta is tender & most broth is soaked up, add cream cheese, milk, and pesto.

8.Stir it & cook over high temp till the cream cheese melts fully.

9.Lastly, add the chopped parmesan and mix it until fully combined.

10.If using, add the spinach & sliced sun-dried tomatoes. Mix until the spinach has wilted, remove pasta from the stove. Decorate pasta with crushed pepper & a pinch of red pepper & serve.

Spinach pesto pasta

Preparation time: 10 minutes
Cooking time: 15 minutes
Servings: 4

Ingredients:

1/2 cup peas
1 whole ripe avocado
2 cups baby spinach leaves
7 tbsp basil pesto
12 oz of fusilli pasta
Salt to taste
1.5 tbsp red wine vinegar
1/2 tsp black pepper

Directions:

1.Cook pasta in boiling water for ten minutes.

2.Transfer the hot pasta over spinach in a bowl.

3.Add pasta liquid to the bowl.

4.Mix vinegar, pepper, peas, pepper, and avocado.
Serve and enjoy it.

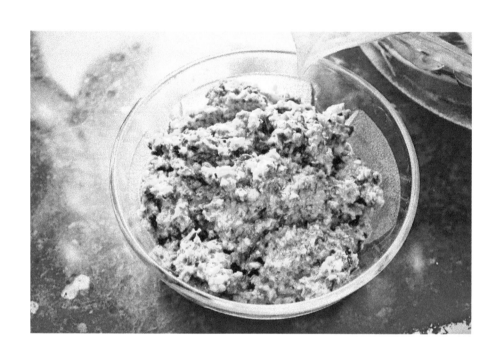

Fiber packed chicken rice

Preparation time: 5 minutes
Cooking time: 10 minutes
Servings: 2

Ingredients:
1 tsp rice vinegar
1 tsp toasted sesame oil
6 scallions root
1 shredded carrot
1 tbsp avocado oil
3 eggs
1 pinch of salt
Black pepper
1/2 cup peas
2 cups cooked brown rice
3 tsp soy sauce
1/2 tsp grated ginger

Directions:

1.Take ½ tbsp of olive oil & heat it.

2.Take eggs in a bowl & whisk until well combined & put a pinch of salt & black pepper powder. Pour these eggs into a saucepan & scramble.

3.Now add half tbsp olive oil in a pan & add scallion & carrots. Sauté the ingredients till they are softened (3-4 min).

4.Take frozen peas in a pan & add rice, vinegar, tamari, ginger & sesame oil. Mix them well. Now turn off the heat & combine with scrambled eggs.

5.Now add salt according to taste.

6. Now cook the whole dish for almost 5-5 min until it is well cooked and warmed.

7.Bean sprouts, veggie & water chestnuts will be a delicious addition to the dish if needed.

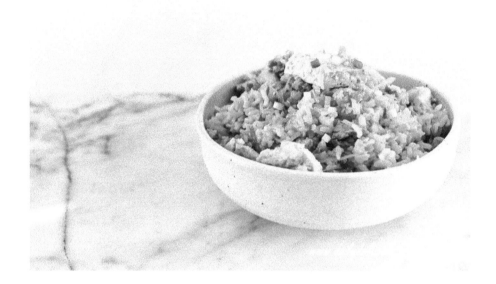

Herb rice

Preparation time: 5 minutes
Cooking time: 20 minutes
Servings: 4

Ingredients:

1 tsp salt
2 Tbsp butter
1 tsp onion black pepper juice
3 cup chicken broth
1 tsp garlic
1/4 cup lemon juice
1.5 cup basmati rice
1/2 tsp rosemary, basil, dill, parsley, oregano, thyme

Directions:

1.Melt butter on moderate heat & add salt & black pepper powder. Keep stirring till the onion is softened.

2.Now add garlic & cook (1 min)

3.Add chicken broth & lemon juice with herb along with rice.

4.Keep stirring until mixed.

5.Now, wait for a boil, cover & lower heat.

6.Keep cooking until rice is well softened & garnish with herbs if required.

7.Serve & enjoy.

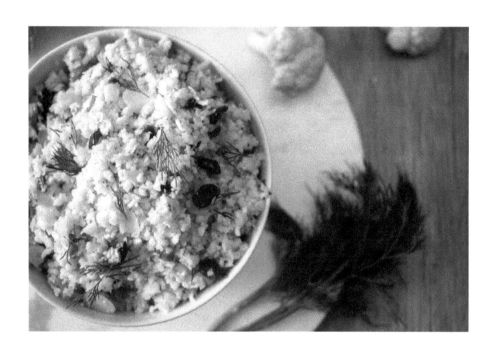

Pecorino pasta with sausage and tomato

Preparation time: 20 minutes
Cooking time: 20 minutes
Servings: 4

Ingredients:

2 tsp olive oil
1 cup sliced onion
8 oz penne
8 oz Italian sausage
6 tbsp grated Romano cheese
1/4 tsp salt
2 tsp garlic
1 1/4 lb tomatoes
1/8 tsp black pepper
1/4 cup torn basil leaves

Directions:

1.Boil & drain pasta.

2.Keep the boiled pasta aside.

3.Now at a full flame, heat a skillet, which should be nonstick.

4.Take oil in a pan & add sausage and onion to it. Cook for about two minutes. Now remove from stove & add pasta, salt, black pepper powder & cheese.

5.Add oil to a pan, swirl to coat.

6.Sprinkle remaining 1/4th cup of cheese and serve

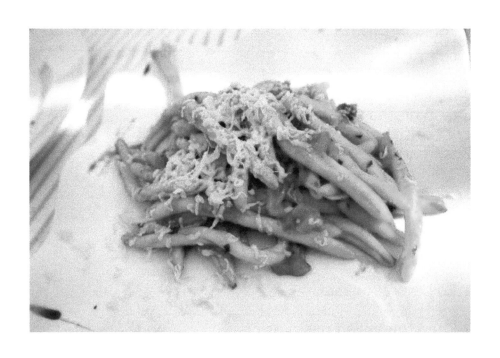

Pesto pasta and shrimp

Preparation time: 10 minutes
Cooking time: 10 minutes
Servings: 3

Ingredients:

10 oz spaghetti
3/4 cup basil pesto
1 lb shrimp
1 tbsp olive oil
1 tsp Italian seasoning
Salt to taste
Black pepper to taste
1/4 cup parmesan cheese

Directions:

1.Bring a pot of salted water to a boil and cook the pasta.

2.While the pasta is cooking, prepare the shrimp. Heat the olive oil in a pan over high heat.

3.Add the shrimp and sprinkle with Italian seasoning, salt, and pepper.

4.Cook for 2-4 minutes or until shrimp is just pink and opaque. Turn off the heat.

5.Drain the pasta and add it to the pan with the shrimp. Stir in the pesto.

6.Add the cherry tomatoes and parmesan cheese to the pan.

7.Garnish with parsley if desired.

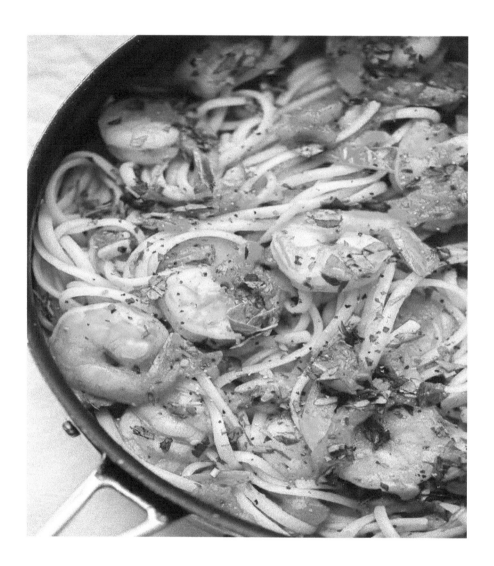

Spanish rice casserole with cheesy beef

Preparation time: 10 minutes
Cooking time: 25 minutes
Servings: 4

Ingredients:

16.8 oz Spanish Rice mix
1 tbsp olive oil
1 red bell pepper
1 cup of corn
1 cup meatless crumbles
1/3 cup sour cream
1/4 cup salsa
1/2 cup Monterey Jack cheese
2 tbsp crumbled queso fresco
1 avocado sliced

Directions:

1.Prepare the rice in a 2.5-liter casserole dish, which should be microwavable.

2.Preheat the microwave up to 375 F.

3.Take a skillet and heat the oil.

4.Now cook bell pepper till tendered 5-7 minutes.

5.Once the rice is cooked, then combine the bell pepper, cooked, meatless crumbles, salsa, sour cream & corn.

6.Now sprinkle the cheese on the top.

7.Bake it, uncovered (10 minutes), till the cheese is melted & browned on top.

8.Top sliced avocado.

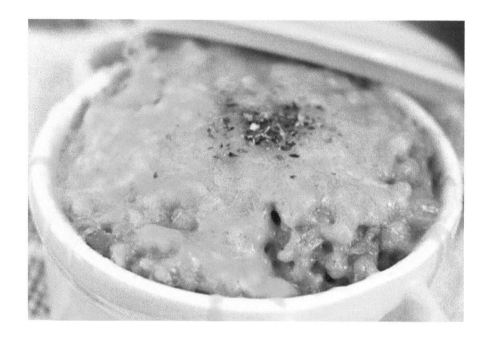

Yangchow Chinese style fried rice

Preparation time: 15 minutes
Cooking time: 20 minutes
Servings: 6

Ingredients:

6 cups cooked white rice
1 cup barbecued pork
1 tsp sugars
1 tsp ginger
10 pieces of shrimps
3/4 cup green peas
1 tsp garlic
1 1/2 tbsp soy sauce
2 tsp salt
1/4 cup green onion
2 beaten eggs
3 tbsp cooking oil

Directions:

1.Heat the oil & sauté ginger-garlic together. Add the shrimps & cook (1 minute).

2.Pour the egg mixture & cook.

3.Divide the cooked egg into pieces.

4.Add rice & soy sauce, salt & sugar, and mix with other ingredients.

5.Add pork, which is barbecued & cook (3 minutes).

6.Add peas & shrimp & cook 3 minutes.

7.Add onions and cook (2 minutes).

8.Turn off heat & transfer to a serving plate.

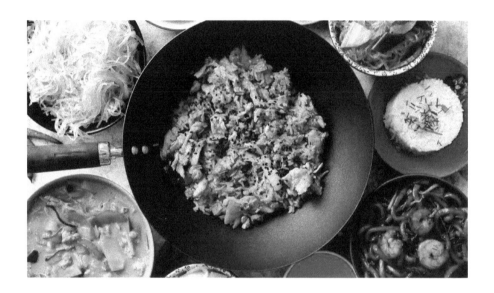

Mahi-mahi pomegranate sauce

Preparation time: 5 minutes
Cooking time: 20 minutes
Servings: 2

Ingredients:

12 oz Mahi-mahi fillets

1/2 cup balsamic vinegar

1/4 cup pomegranate juice
1 tbsp olive oil
1 tbsp squeezed lemon juice
1/2 cup pomegranate seeds

Directions:

1.Preheat microwave up to 450 deg.

2.Take baking dish & lay Mahi fillets, drizzle with lemon juice & olive oil.

3.Bake it for 15-20 minutes

4.Take a pan & heat vinegar, pomegranate juice & seeds over high heat.

5.Bring a boil & let the sauce to reduce (20 minutes)

6.Spoon the fillets.

7.Serve & enjoy.

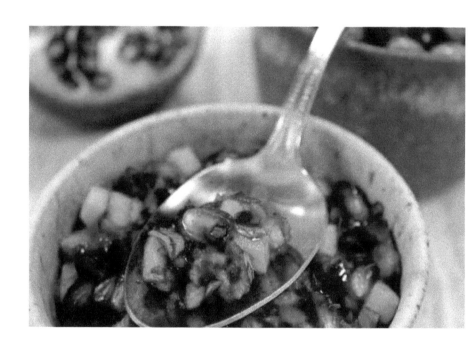

Feta tomato sea bass

Preparation time: 10 minutes
Cooking time: 10 minutes
Servings: 4

Ingredients:

2 oz dry white wine
2 tbsp lemon juice
32 oz sea bass fillets
4 oz feta cheese
5 ripe tomatoes
5 tbsp olive oil
2 tbsp butter
2 tbsp basil
3 garlic cloves
1 tbsp oregano
Salt & pepper

Directions:

1.Take fish & rub salt & pepper over it.

2.Heat the pan & add olive oil.

3.Put the fish in a pan.

4.Cook it until it is golden brown.

5.Add basil, cheese, lemon juice, tomatoes & garlic.

6.Bake 12-15 minutes at 400 deg. Take the dish out and finish it with butter.

7.The dish is ready.

8.Now serve and enjoy.

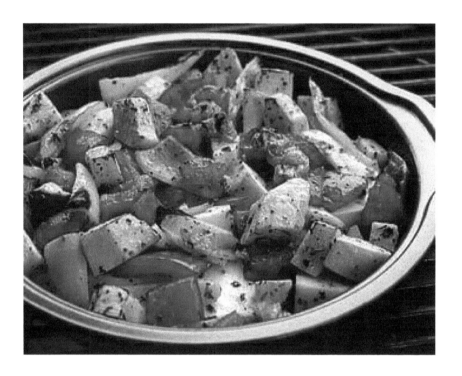

Crab stew

Preparation time: 25 minutes
Cooking time: 25 minutes
Servings: 4

Ingredients:

2 tbsp sweet paprika
1/2 cup heavy cream
6 tbsp unsalted butter
1/4 lb shrimp
1 lb lump crabmeat
2 cups steamed rice
3/4 tsp chipotle Chile powder
2 tbsp all-purpose flour
1/4 cup dry sherry
2 cups clam juice
1 cup of water
1 small onion
1 garlic clove
Salt and pepper
1 tbsp leaf parsley

Directions:

1.Melt one tbsp of butter in a pan.

2.Add shrimp & cook at moderate heat. Now add sherry & cook for 2 minutes.

3.Add clam juice & water.

4.Bring a boil & simmer moderately at low heat for 10 minutes.

5.Strain broth. Now again, melt 2 tbsp butter in the pan.

6.Add garlic & onion & cook at moderate heat till it is softened.
7.Add paprika & chipotle, stirring for 3 minutes. Now stir with flour.

8.Whisk broth in the pan. Cook till it becomes smooth & then bring a boil.

9.Simmer at low heat. Whisk till it is just thickened 5 minutes.

10Add cream, simmer & season with salt & pepper.

11.Take a skillet & melt 3 tbsp butter.

12.Now gently stir the crab & cook at moderate heat.

13. Toss for a few minutes' till warmed 4 minutes.

14.Season with salt & pepper, Spoon steamed rice into the shallow bowls, Ladle shellfish sauce on rice & top with crab. Sprinkle with parsley & serve.

Savory zucchini loaf

Preparation time: 25 min
Cooking time: 50-55 min
Servings: 8

Ingredients:

5 tbsp of olive oil
1 small, diced zucchini.
Half cup of hazelnuts.
¾ cup of tomato (sun-dried).
Half cup milk
1 cup all-purpose flour.
3 eggs
2 tsp of baking powder
2/3 cup of mozzarella cheese.
¼ cup of basil.
¼ tbsp of black pepper
¼ tbsp of sea salt

Directions:

1.Preheat the microwave up to 350 F

2.Toast hazelnuts on moderate heat in a frypan. Sauté diced zucchini on medium heat (5 min).

3.Place tomatoes in a bowl. For ten minutes, cover it with hot water. Drain it and place it aside.

4.Take three eggs and whisk them in a bowl.

5.Add milk to eggs & beat.

6. Add flour & baking soda mix until it becomes smooth.

7.Add 5 tbsp of olive oil & pepper.
8.Mix it well.

9.Add other ingredients tomatoes, basil, hazelnuts & mozzarella. Mix delicately with a spatula.

10.Spray the pan with cooking spray & pour the batter into it.

11.Bake for almost 45 min until toothpick comes out dry and clean.

12.Cut it into slices & serve.

Chilled Pea and mint soup

Prep time: 20 min
Cook time: 20-25 min
Servings: 4

Ingredients:

2 tbsp of butter
1 chopped onion medium size.
2 cups of water.
2 pounds of frozen green peas.
2 cups of vegetable broth.
¼ cup of fresh mint leaves
¼ cup of fresh parsley
1 tsp of fresh lemon juice.
Half tsp cayenne.
Mint leaves for garnishing

Directions:

1.Melt the butter in a large pan.

2.Add onions & cook till softened for 7 minutes.

3. Combine vegetable stock & water in a medium-sized saucepan.

4.Stir in 1/2 of the water mixture in the large pan along with the onions. Increase the heat & bring to boil.

5.Add peas & bring to a boil for one minute.

6.Remove from stove.

7.Add remaining water mixture with the mint, parsley & cayenne.

8.Puree with an immersion blender in a pot till it becomes smooth.

9.Season using lime juice.

10.Cool until chilled.

11.Serve in the bowls with mint leaves.

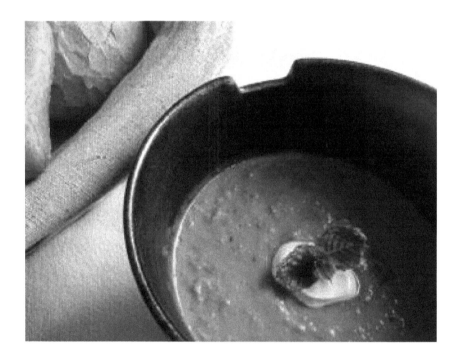

Watermelon & cantaloupe salad

Preparation time: 10 minutes
Cooking time: 0 minute
Servings: 6

Ingredients:

¼ cup of pine nuts
2 cups of diced cantaloupe,
6 cups of diced watermelon.
5 tbsp of olive oil
2/3 cup of crumbled feta cheese.
1/4 cup of fresh mint.
¼ tsp of black pepper powder.

Directions:

1.Toast pine nuts in a pan.

2.Add olive oil, cantaloupe & watermelon in a bowl.

3.Sprinkle the cheese, mint & pepper.

4.Mix it delicately.

5. Chill for one hour.

6.Serve.

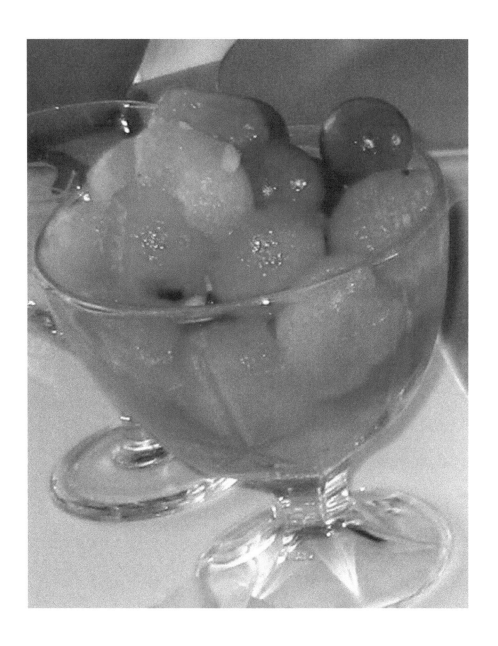

Southern-fried okra

Preparation time: 5 min
Cooking time: 25 min
Servings: 6

INGREDIENTS

Half cup flour-unbleached
Half cup of cornmeal.
1/8th tsp of salt
1/4th tsp of fresh black pepper
1 egg.
2 tbsp of milk
1/3rd cup of sunflower oil
3 cups of fresh okra

Directions:

1.Preheat the microwave up to 300 F

2.Mix & whisk together the flour, salt, black pepper & cayenne in a bowl.

3.Beat egg & milk in a bowl.

4.Heat sunflower oil.

5.Dip okra pieces in the egg batter & roll in a mixture.

6.Fry in the pan. Turn over after two min.

7.Remove the cooked okra with a spoon & drain each batch.

8.Transfer 1st batch to a baking dish to keep it warm while the remaining okra is cooking.

9.Place the 2nd batch of the fried okra in the oven till the final batch is done.

10.Serve it immediately.

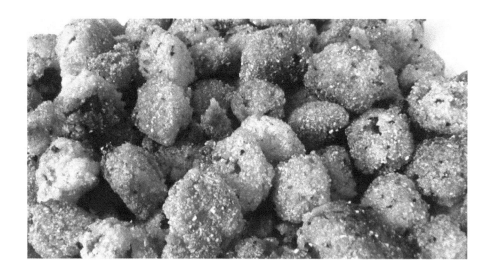

Pesto Pasta with Peas and Mozzarella

Preparation time: 10 minutes
Cooking time: 0 minute
Servings: 3

Ingredients:
2 cups green peas
1 cup mozzarella balls low sodium
4 cups Boiled Penna Pasta
2 cups fresh basil leaves
¼ tsp Garlic powder
1 tbsp Lemon juice
2 tsp zest of a lemon
1/3 cup olive oil
¼ tsp Salt
¼ tsp Pepper

Directions:

1.For making pesto, add all the ingredients in a blender or food processor and mix them except for olive oil. Pulse until crudely sliced.

2.Reduce the food processor's speed or blender, slowly add olive oil to it, mix it well, and blend. Scrape down the sides of the food processor/blender to fully mix the end. Add salt & pepper.

3.Add mozzarella, pasta, and peas into a large bowl. Add pesto according to requirement Add pesto as desired and then mix all ingredients.

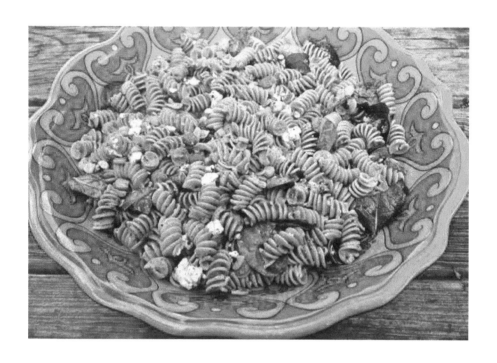

Balsamic Roasted Green Beans

Preparation time: 5 minutes
Cooking time: 17 minutes
Servings: 1 cup

Ingredients:

1 lb Green beans
2 Chopped Garlic Cloves
1 tbsp Balsamic vinegar
1 tbsp Olive oil
⅛ tsp Salt
⅛ tsp Pepper

Directions:

1.Preheat oven to 425°F.

2.Mix green beans along with olive oils, pepper & salt in a large bowl.

3.Evenly spread green beans on a foil or parchment paper-lined on a baking sheet.

4.Bake them for 10-12 mints in the oven until it turns light brown

5.Spread garlic with green beans & mix well to combine. Then again, bake it for another 5 minutes till beans are warm & browned.

6.Remove from oven & toss with balsamic vinegar.

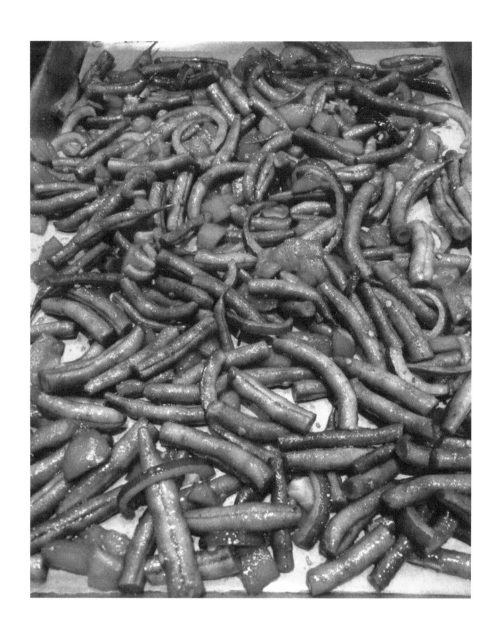

Mac in a Flash (Macaroni and Cheese)

Preparation time: 2 minutes
Cooking time: 10 minutes
Servings: 4

Ingredients:

3 cups Water
1 cup Noodles
½ cup Grated Cheddar Cheese
1 tsp Butter
⅛ tsp dry mustard

Directions:

1.Add noodles in boiling water, boil it for 5 to 7 minutes or until tender, and then drain the boiled noodles.

2.Sprinkle the grated cheddar cheese on the hot noodles & mix it with butter and dry grounded mustard

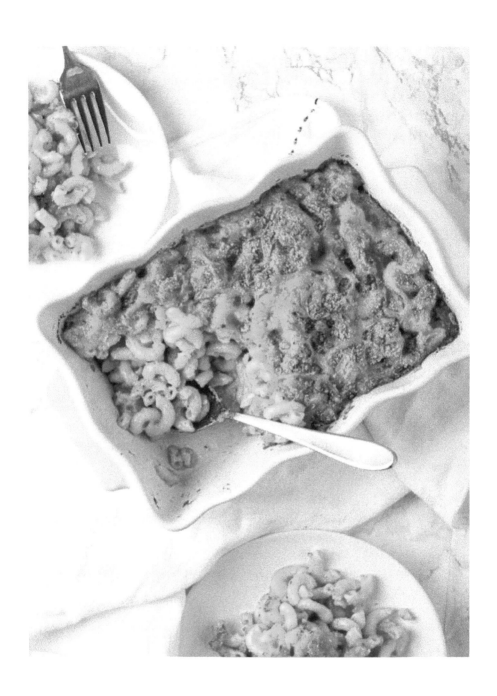

Costa Rican Gallo Pinto

Preparation time: 5 minutes
Cooking time: 30 minutes
Servings: 4

Ingredients:

1/3 cup dry black beans
4 tbsp Olive oil
110g Chopped Onion
2 Chopped Garlic Cloves
1 chopped red bell pepper
1 tsp Cumin
1 tbsp Salsa Lizano
3 cups Cooked White rice
½ tsp black pepper
Bit of smoked paprika
¼ cup Chopped Cilantro
4 Hard-boiled eggs
Salt to taste

Directions:

Preparation of beans advance

1.Soak black beans in one and a half cups of water at least for 2 hrs. or overnight.

2.Add beans in boiling water and boil them until beans tender for ten- fifteen. Save beans along with water.

Preparation for Gallo pinto

1.Take a large frying pan and heat the oil over medium heat.

2.Then add sliced veggies (garlic, onion, & red pepper) to it.

3.Fry and stir it while frying unless or until vegies becomes soft & aromatic.
4.After adding cumin and salsa Lozano in it, mix, then gin cook gin for two to three more minutes.

5.Now mix the boiled bens and its water in it and again cook for just one mint.

6.Combine the cooked rice & make sure that stir until rice is completely mixed with the beans.

7.Cover the frying pan, reduce the heat & cook again for one to two minutes, till the rice is warmed.

8.Flavor with smoked paprika, pepper & cilantro for good flavor.

9.Finally, add this to a bowl and decorate it with a hard-boiled egg on top.

Cheese Quiche

Preparation time: 5 minutes
Cooking time: 45 minutes
Servings: 8

Ingredients:

4 Marginally beaten eggs
Splash of Pepper
1.5 cup milk
3 oz shredded cheddar cheese
¼ cup Chopped onion
1 tsp Parsley leaves Pastry shell un-baked

Directions:

1.Preheat0oven to 350°F.

2.Mix all ingredients in a large bowl & mix it perfectly.

3.Now add already prepared unbaked pastry shell.

4.Bake this for forty to forty-five minutes.

5.Cut into eight slices but cool this before baking.

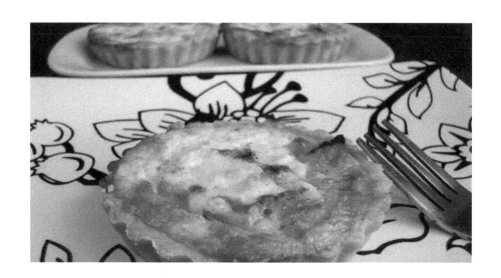

Cheesy thyme waffles

Preparation time: 10 minutes
Cooking time: 7 minutes
Servings: 2

Ingredients:

2 eggs
1/3 cup parmesan cheese
1 tsp garlic powder
1 tsp thyme
1 cup collard greens
1 tbsp olive oil
2 stalks onion
1/2 cauliflower
1/2 tsp salt
1 cup shredded mozzarella cheese
1 tbsp of sesame seeds
1/2 tsp black pepper

Directions:

1.Cut cauliflower & slice onions.

2.Add cauliflower to the blender.

3.Add onions, thyme & collard greens to the blender &
pulse again.

4.Now add the processed mixture to a bowl.

5.Mix it well to form a smooth batter.

6.A heat waffle iron.

7.Pour the mixture into the waffle iron, ensuring that it is spread properly.

8.Cook well & serve hot.

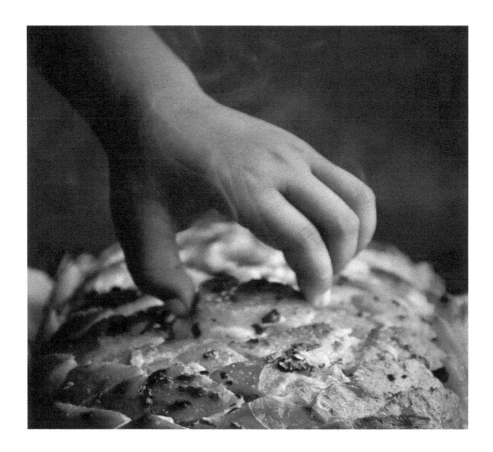

Baked egg and asparagus with cheese parmesan

Preparation time: 10minutes
Cooking time: 15minutes
Servings: 3

Ingredients:

30 spears asparagus
6 eggs
3 tbsp parmesan cheese
3/4 tsp salt
3 tsp butter
3 tsp olive oil
3/4 tsp black pepper

Directions:

1.Preheat microwave up to 400 deg.

2.Take a small pot of water.

3.Add salt & add asparagus.

4.Stir it well.

5.When water boils again, please remove it from the stove.

6.Drain asparagus & transfer it to a bowl filled with cold water.

7.Distribute asparagus.

8.Among three baking dishes, Top center of the baking dish along with one tsp of butter. Season with salt.

9.Add eggs to the baking dish.
10.Bake for 10 min.

11.Remove it from the microwave.

12.Top each portion with cheese & black pepper.

13.Return to microwave & bake it for 7 min.

14.Serve and enjoy.

Creamy cold salad

Preparation time: 10 minutes
Cooking time: 1 minute
Servings: 3

Ingredients:

8 oz salad macaroni
1/4 sliced green onion
1/2 cup red pepper
1/2 cup black olives
1 cup broccoli florets
1/2 cup cucumber

Dressing

1/2 cup mayonnaise
2 tsp vinegar
1/2 tsp kosher salt
1/2 tsp black pepper
1/2 tsp sugar

Directions:

1.Cook pasta.

2.When noodles are cooked, add broccoli.

3.Let broccoli boil 40 sec.

4.Drain everything.

5.Rinse well

6.Stir with mayonnaise, salt, pepper, vinegar & sugar in a bowl.

7.Add cooked pasta & broccoli in a bowl & stir well.
8.Add cucumber, olives, pepper, & onion.

9.Stir again.

10.Cover & refrigerate until the ready dish is ready to serve.

11.Stir again before serving.

12.Enjoy the food!

Peppy pepper tomato salad

Preparation time: 5 minutes
Cooking time: 10 minutes
Servings: 4

Ingredients:
One small garlic
1/4 cup olive oil
1 tbsp sherry vinegar
1 tsp balsamic vinegar
Salt and pepper
1 pound tomatoes
1.5 pounds red peppers,
1 tbsp basil
1 leaf lettuce

Directions:

1.Dressing: mix sherry vinegar, garlic, olive oil, balsamic vinegar, salt, and black pepper powder according to taste.

2.Cut roasted peppers strips.

3.Toss with dressing.

4.Add 1/2 basil & toss again.

5.Remove & discard tough outer leaves.

6.Wash & dry the leaves & tear them to pieces.

7.Toss with tomatoes & dressing & basil.

8.Line platter.

9.Top with peppers.

10.Serve slightly chilled.

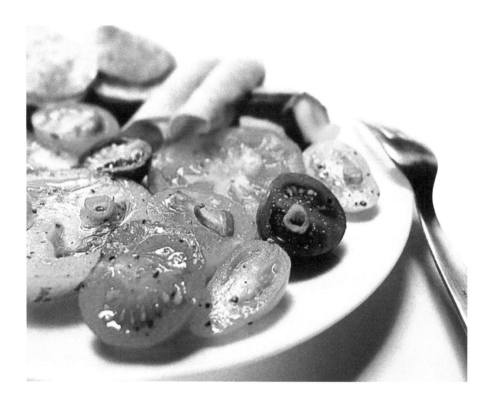

Spinach and grilled feta salad

Preparation time: 10 minutes
Cooking time: 20 minutes
Servings: 1

Ingredients:

1/2 tbsp olive oil
1 oz feta cheese
1 cup shredded mozzarella cheese
1 pinch of salt
Pepper to taste
1 clove garlic
2 ciabatta rolls
1/4 lb spinach

Directions:

1.Mince garlic & add to a pan with olive oil.

2.Cook at moderate heat for 3 minutes.

3.Add frozen spinach & turn heat up.

4.Cook 5 minutes.

5.Season it lightly with sea salt & black pepper.

6.Cut rolls in half.

7.Add shredded mozzarella & half oz. of feta to bottom

8.Divide cooked spinach.

9.Then top each sandwich with a pinch of red pepper plus more mozzarella.

10.Place top of ciabatta roll on sandwiches & transfer in a non- stick pan

11.Fill the pot with water for creating weight.

12.Place pot on the top of sandwiches to press them.

13.Flip sandwiches carefully.

14. Place the weighted pot on top & cook.

15.Serve hot and enjoy.

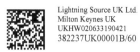

Lightning Source UK Ltd.
Milton Keynes UK
UKHW020633190421
382237UK00001B/60

9 781802 690279